Concepts of Comprehensive Laboratory Diagnostic Methods for Viral Hepatitis Markers of Infection of Public Health Importance

Adeleye Solomon Bakarey
Inioluwa Oyindamola Akinboade
Yetunde Adebisi Aken'Ova

ELIVA PRESS

ELIVA PRESS

Adeleye Solomon Bakarey
Inioluwa Oyindamola Akinboade
Yetunde Adebisi Aken'Ova

This book describes the Concepts of Comprehensive Laboratory Diagnostic Methods for Viral Hepatitis Markers of Infection of Public Health Importance. It will serve as a guide for medical scientists, undergraduate and postgraduate medicos and allied medical professional in various higher institutions worldwide especially in developing countries where viral hepatitis is endemic. It simplifies the diagnostic methods used with ease of understanding so as to relieve the burden experienced by scientists in the field of medicine, microbiology and general science. The medical laboratory scientists, Nurses, Doctors, residents, house officers and their lecturers will also find the book useful as a guide for teaching and learning.

This book has been developed as a guide to laboratory diagnostic methods for viral hepatitis useful for students of medicine, medical microbiology, medical residents, medical laboratory science/scientists, nurses, doctors and other allied medical professionals. It is designed to provide any aforementioned category of students a concise presentation of the important and most relevant aspects of laboratory diagnostic methods for viral hepatitis with many markers of infection such as HBV of medical importance and to unravel the diseases they cause. The diagnostic methods have been simplified and formatted for easy understanding of all medical laboratorians and as a quick revision for professional examination in medicine and medical microbiology.

The book contains two disease investigation procedures with relevant guidelines and also serves as a guide for manuscript writing for all researchers in medical microbiology and allied sciences. It will also help scientific investigations that require systemic arrangement of ideas for which the end products will be beneficial to mankind. I hope all readers of this book will find the information contained therein useful.

Published: Eliva Press SRL
Address: MD-2060, bd.Cuza-Voda, 1/4, of. 21 Chişinău, Republica Moldova
Email: info@elivapress.com
Website: www.elivapress.com

ISBN: 978-1-952751-31-8

Transmission Transmissible Hepatitis B Virus Markers Of Infection Among Sickle Cell Disease Patients Receiving Care At A Tertiary Health Facility In Ibadan, Southwest Nigeria*

[1,2]*Bakarey A. S., [1]Akinboade I. O., [3]Aken'ova Y. A..

[1]Department of Biomedical Laboratory Science, College of Medicine, University of Ibadan, Ibadan, Nigeria

[2]Institute for Advanced Medical Research and Training, College of Medicine, University of Ibadan, Ibadan, Nigeria

[3]Department of Haematology, College of Medicine, University of Ibadan, Ibadan, Nigeria

*Correspondence: Dr. A. S. Bakarey
Institute for Advanced Medical Research and Training, College of Medicine, University College Hospital, University of Ibadan, Ibadan, Nigeria. Postal code: 200212, Queen Elizabeth II Road, Ibadan, Nigeria.

Abstract

Introduction: Hepatitis B virus infection attacks the liver and can cause both acute and chronic disease. Sickle cell disease (SCD) patients are at risk of transmission transmissible viral hepatitis due to their constant need for blood transfusion. However, these patients could have been infected with HBV but may not know their status due to asymptomatic nature of the infection. Therefore this study was designed to determine the burden of HBV markers of infection among SCD patients attending the Haematology clinic at a tertiary health facility in Ibadan, Nigeria.

Methodology: A cross-sectional study was investigated among 112 consenting SCD patients (M=45; F=67) age ranged 15-60years (Mean age=26.9; Mean PCV=24±4.8) attending Haematology clinic at the University College Hospital,

1

*Adeleye Solomon Bakarey, Inioluwa Oyindamola Akinboade & Yetunde Adebisi Aken'Ova (2018) Transmission transmissible hepatitis B virus markers of infection among sickle cell disease patients receiving care at a tertiary health facility in Ibadan, southwest Nigeria, Journal of Immunoassay and Immunochemistry, 39:4, 416-427, DOI: 10.1080/15321819.2018.1495649

Ibadan. A structured questionnaire was administered to capture demographic and other relevant information. Blood samples from each participant were tested for HBV markers by ELISA technique while data were analyzed using SPSS version 21 with p< 0.05 considered significant.

Results: A total of 5(4.5%), 0(0%) and 15(13.4%) were positive for HBsAg, HBeAg and HBeAb respectively. Also, 63(56.3%) of the participants have never been transfused while 49(43.8%) had received blood transfusion at a point in time. No significant difference (p=0.095) found for prevalence of HBV markers among those that had received blood transfusion and those that did not. Highest rates for HBsAg (3.6%) and HBeAb (10.7%) were observed among female than their male (HBsAg (0.9%) and HBeAb (2.8%) counterparts (p=0.065). No significant associations (p>0.05) among those with incisions, sexually active and the vaccinated individuals for HBV markers. There was a significant difference (p=0.025) among the married participants for HBeAb with higher HBeAb rate (64.3%).

Conclusion: This study reported high rates of HBV markers of infection among SCD patients. It is therefore advocated that donated blood must pass through rigorous screening processes before it is transfused.

Keywords: HBV markers, Sickle cell disease, Transfusion transmissible infection, Haematology, Ibadan.

Introduction

Hepatitis B virus (HBV) is a major cause of morbidity and mortality in sub-Sahara Africa and it is known to be endemic in Africa resulting in both acute and chronic liver diseases [1]. It infects every member of the population which doesn't exclude sickle cell patients and it is transmitted through contact with the blood and other body fluids of an infected person [2]. The virus has a double stranded DNA and it is of the family of *Hepadnaviridae* [3]. The viral particle consists of an outer lipid envelope and an icosahedral nucleoplasmid core composed of protein which encloses the viral DNA and polymerase enzyme [4-5]. An estimated 257 million people are living with hepatitis B virus infection with about 50 million chronic carriers in Africa [2].

Sickle cell disease occurs when an individual inherits two abnormal copies of the haemoglobin gene which is on chromosome 11 [6-7]. It results in an abnormality in the oxygen carrying pigment of the blood which is haemoglobin in the erythrocytes which leads to a rigid sickle cell shape of the red cell [6]. About 4.4 million people have sickle cell disease as at 2015 and 80% of the cases occur in sub-Sahara Africa [8-9]. It resulted in about 114,800 deaths in the same year [9].

The first modern report of sickle cell disease was in 1846 from the autopsy of an executed run-away slave Lebby, [6,10]. Sickle cell disease raises the chance of infection with HBV [11]. Sickle cell patient having the hepatitis infection have very similar traits to those without sickle cell haemoglobinpathies-which include; liver cirrhosis, hepatocellular carcinoma and the risk of pancreatic cancer- except severe hyperbilirubineamia. This hyperbilirubinamia occurs as a result of increase load of red cell breakdown products due to the continuous hemolysis [4].

The seroprevalence of hepatitis B surface antigen (HBsAg) among sickle cell anemia children was 17.3% [1]. HBV is of high interest in sickle cell anemia patients because they are chronic blood recipients as a result of frequent anemia. They are, therefore, potentially at high risk of HBV infection [12]. Patients with sickle cell anaemia in Nigeria have tendencies to visit traditional healers who administer scarifications and ritual marks that may expose them to HBV infection as well [13]. Hepatitis B serological markers are; Hepatitis B surface antigen (HBsAg) which is a protein on the surface of the hepatitis B virus (HBV); it can be detected in the serum during acute or chronic HBV infection [14]. The presence of HBsAg indicates that the person has hepatitis B infection.

According Akinbami *et al.* [15], Total hepatitis B core antibody (anti-HBc) appears at the onset of symptoms in acute hepatitis B infection and persists for life. The presence of anti-HBc indicates previous or ongoing infection with HBV. Immunoglobulin M (IgM) antibody to hepatitis B core antigen (IgM anti-HBc) and its presence usually indicates acute (<6 months) as opposed to chronic hepatitis B infection [16]. It can also be found during viral reactivations. Hepatitis B e antigen (HBeAg) is a product of the nucleocapsid (envelope) gene of the hepatitis B virus that is found in serum during acute and chronic hepatitis B infection. Its presence indicates that the virus is replicating and the infected person has high levels of HBV [17]. However patients that are HBeAg negative may also have high levels of HBV [18-19]. Hepatitis B e antibody (HBeAb or anti-HBe) Spontaneous conversion from e antigen to e antibody (a change known as "e" seroconversion) is a predictor of long- term clearance of HBV in patients undergoing antiviral therapy and indicates lower levels of HBV. Spontaneous "e" seroconversion also occurs in natural infection. Hepatitis B surface antibody (anti-HBs) is generally interpreted as indicating recovery and immunity from HBV infection. Anti-HBs also develops in a person who has been successfully vaccinated against hepatitis B [20-21].

Sickle cell patients are at risk of blood borne infections such as viral hepatitis due to their need for regular blood transfusion. This together with the asymptomatic nature of the hepatitis B infection has made it important for sickle cell patients to be tested for the presence of the hepatitis markers in their serum [8]. Furthermore, a lot of these sickle cell anaemia patients are totally unaware of their predisposition to the hepatitis B infection due to the above stated fact. This study aims at enlightening them as regards this pertinent issue. Due to this wide knowledge gap, sickle cell anaemia patients have the tendency visit traditional healers who administer scarifications and ritual marks that may expose them to HBV infection. Although other studies [1,12] have been carried out on HBV only among children and a narrow age range sickle cell patients in Nigeria, however, this present study was aimed at determining this infection among adults with a wider age range sickle cell patients with a view at estimating the burden in southwest Nigeria. Therefore this study was designed to determine the burden of HBV markers of infection among sickle cell patients attending the Haematology clinic at a tertiary health facility in Ibadan, southwest Nigeria.

Methodology

Study design: This is a cross sectional study to determine the prevalence of hepatitis B infection among sickle cell patients attending the haematology clinic at the University College Hospital Ibadan Nigeria.

Study location: This study was conducted at the Haematology day care unit, University College Hospital Ibadan Nigeria. University College Hospital is a Federal teaching hospital affiliated to the University Of Ibadan. It was established in the year 1948 having only two departments at the time. Since its establishment, the institution has trained over 60,000 doctors, 501 dentists, 4,513 nurses, 1062 laboratory scientists and many other health professionals. Presently, it offers postgraduate training in Internal Medicine, Surgery Obstetrics and Gyneacology, Pediatrics, Otorhinolaryngology, Anesthesia, Laboratory Medicine Which Includes Haematology, Psychiatry, Community Medicine, Radiology and Dentistry. It has

850 bed spaces with 163 examination couches. it has about 60 departments presently which includes the haematology departments.

Study Population: The target population is sickle cell anaemic patients between the ages fifteen and sixty attending the haematology clinic at University College Hospital in the North. A cross sectional study was carried out among112 sickle cell anaemia patients' age ranged 15 and 60 years. The participants included 45 males (40.2%) and 67(59.8) females. The mean PCV of the participants was 24 ± 4.8 with 11(11.0%) of them had PCV ≤ 18 and 89 (89%) had PCV ≥ 18. 49(56.3%) people didn't receive blood transfusion while 63(56.3%) had previously received blood transfusion.

Enrolment of participants

A total of 112 consenting participants (M=45, F=67; age ranged 15-60 years and median age=26.4 years) were enrolled for the study beweent August and October, 2017. The study relied upon availability of participants with sickle cell anaemia who came for medical checkup and others on admission at the Haematology clinic at University College Hospital, Ibadan. Health education messages relating to HBV prevalence and prevention were provided to each prospective participant prior to their enrolment in the study. Subsequently, a structured questionnaire was used to capture the socio-demographic information of the target population. Blood sample was collected from each consenting participant by a trained phlebotomist. Ethical approval for the study was granted by the UI/UCH Ethics Committee with assigned number (UI/EC/17/0319). All the participants were well informed on the nature, purpose and processes involved in the study prior to their enrolment. Participation was voluntary while the non-consenting participants were excluded from the study thereby maintaining the principle of autonomy. Verbal consent was used to enroll the participants into the study. Confidentiality, privacy and

6

anonymity of the information for each participant were guaranteed for the sample provided.

Sample collection

Five milliliters (5ml) of blood sample was collected from each person by venepuncture into a sterile EDTA specimen labeled bottle with the subject's laboratory identity number and date of collection. The labeled bottle with specimen was temporarily kept in rack placed in Jablow box containing cold iced pack and taken to IAMRAT laboratory, University College Hospital Ibadan Nigeria where the plasma was extracted from whole blood by centrifugation at 2000rpm for 20minutes. The extracted plasma was separated into three aliquots immediately to prevent haemolysis. They were stored at −20°C until lab analysis was carried out at the Institute for Advanced Medical Research and Training, College of Medicine, University of Ibadan, Ibadan, Nigeria. An aliquot of the plasma specimen was used for the detection of HBV serological markers of infection, while the other aliquots and the red cells were stored as reference samples in the same institute ultra-low freezers.

ELISA test for HBV markers

All 112 samples were screened for HBsAg, HBeAg, anti-HBe using Enzyme Linked Immunosorbent Assay (ELISA) test kits (MELSIN Hepatitis B virus surface Antigen ELISA kit, Hepatitis B virus e Antigen ELISA Kit and Antibody to Hepatitis B virus e Antigen kit were used to perform the tests with numbers; cat#: MID-003 , 006 and 007 respectively). All assays were carried out in line with the manufacturer's instructions. The optical density was read using the Emax endpoint ELISA microplate reader (Molecular Devices, California, USA) and the results interpreted accordingly.

Results

The ages of the 112 participants ranged from 15-60years with mean value 30.4±11.1 years. The participants included 45 males (40.2%) and 67(59.8) females of which 87(77.7%) and 25(22.3%) of them had HbSS and HbSC haemoglobin phenotypes respectively. The participants were made up of 37 (37%) married people and 55(55%) single ones in with 88(80%) of persons from the Yoruba, 5(4.5%) from Hausa and 17(15.5%) from Igbo tribes respectively. Seventy two (67.9%) of them had tertiary education as their highest level of education while 24(22.6%) and 10(9.4%) had secondary and primary/informal levels of education respectively (Tables 1).

Overall prevalence rates of 5(4.5%), 0(0%) and 15(13.4%) were found for HBsAg, HBeAg and HBeAb respectively. The mean PCV of the participants was 24 ± 4.8 with 13(11.6%) of them had PCV ≤18 and 99 (88.4%) had PCV ≥ 18. 49(56.3%) people didn't receive blood transfusion while 63(56.3%) had previously received blood transfusion indicating that 63(56.3%) participants had never been transfused while 49(43.8%) had received blood transfusion at a point in time. There was no significant difference in the prevalence of the markers of viral infection among those that had received blood transfusion and those that did not (p > 0.05) (Table 2).

Seventy two (66.1%) participants had prior knowledge of hepatitis B virus while 37(33.9%) were ignorant with 8(7.4%) having family history of the virus while 99 (91.7%) did not have such history. Ninety seven (90.6%) of them had no incisions on their bodies while 10 (9.4%) were incised at one point in their lives. The participants that have been previously vaccinated were 26(24.8%) while 79(75.2%) had not been previously vaccinated. A total of 8(7.3%) individuals had multiple sexual partners and 102(92.7%) had one or no sexual partner. However, none of these variables were statistically significant (p>0.05) (Table 3).

The highest positivity (64.3%) for immunity against the transmission transmissible HBeAg was observed among female participants. No significant difference was observed among those with incision\s, sexually active ones and the vaccinated individuals for the viral markers. There was a significant association (p=0.025) among the married participants for HBeAb of which the single and unmarried ones having lower seropositivity (Table 4)

Discussion

In past years, sickle cell patients have been reported to be prone to transmission transmissible viral infections because of their constant need for blood transfusion which is as a result of their chronic anaemia [12]. This study found a prevalence rate of 4.5% for HBsAg (table 2) which is higher than 2.4% reported by Bolarinwa et al. [22] which may be due to the sensitivity of diagnostic technique used. Their study was carried out using the rapid kit contrary to the ELISA kit used in this study which is more sensitive. It is also higher than that reported Samuel et al. [23] in Ghana (3.5%) which is perhaps due to difference in geographical location and their higher sample size.

Furthermore, a previous study found a prevalence of 3.6% in Ghana which was lower than what was obtained in this study and didn't attribute it to blood transfusion but rather sexual activity of the study group (10-18) years [24]. This therefore indicates that blood transfusion may not have direct relationship with HBV transmission as noted in this study (p>0.05). Hepatitis B virus is a major cause of morbidity and mortality in sub-Sahara Africa and it is known to be endemic in Africa [1,16]. An estimated 257 million people are living with hepatitis

B virus infection with about 50 million chronic carriers in Africa [2]. This was established by Ampofo *et al.* [25] in Ghana that recorded a prevalence of 18% among blood donors. The lower rate found in this study is perhaps due to rigorous screening process put in place for before blood is transfused [26].

Hepatitis B surface Antigen (HBsAg) is the first detectable viral antigen to appear during infection. However, early in an infection, this antigen may not be present and it may be undetectable later in the infection as it is being cleared by the host [17]. Shortly after the appearance of the HBsAg, another antigen called hepatitis B e antigen (HBeAg) will appear. Traditionally, the presence of HBeAg in a host's serum is associated with much higher rates of viral replication and enhanced infectivity [19]. During the natural course of an infection, the HBeAg may be cleared, and antibodies to the 'e' antigen (anti-HBe) will arise immediately afterwards [18,27], this is why they were used in this study as markers of infection.

The prevalence of HBeAb was 13.4% and that of the corresponding antigen, HBeAg was 0%. The presence of HBeAb and the absence of HBeAg has described as seroconversion and attributed to clearance of the virus and decline in viral replication in a previous study [18] but other findings have identified these parameters among active carriers [22,28]. In lieu of this, further investigation, particularly at the genetic level is required to differentiate between the active and inactive carriers in this category. A significant difference (p=0.025) was observed among the single (unmarried) participants of this study. It was observed that they had a higher prevalence of the markers than the married ones. Thus, it can perhaps be attributed to their lifestyle and the fact that they may not be committed to a particular sexual partner. This has further demonstrated the relationship of HBV transmission with risky lifestyle as earlier reported [29-30].

In this study, there was no significant difference (p=0.346) between the prevalence of the viral markers among male and female even though female participants were observed to have a higher seropositivity (Table 4). This could be attributed to the higher preponderance of females in this study compared to that of male counterparts. This is in agreement with an earlier finding which reported that equal number of males and females were tested and there was no significant difference between them [23]. It was also established by Bolarinwa *et al.,*[22] which found no significant difference in seropositivity among male and their female counterparts indicating that there was no gender bias for HBV infection in this study.

Conclusion

This study has identified high rates and circulation of HBV markers of infection among sickle cell anaemia patients indicating that they are high risk population group. There was no significant difference in seropositivity among those transfused and those that were not as well as the different age groups and sex. This could be attributed to the rigorous screening process donated blood passes through before it is transfused. A significant difference was however observed between the seropositivity of viral markers among single and married participants and can be attributed tip differences in lifestyle.

References

1. Baba J., Jiya NM., Ahmed H. Prevalence of Hepatitis B Surface Antigen In Children With Sickle Cell Anaemia. Sahel Med J 2014; 17:15-8 March 2014

2. World Health Organisation. Epidemiological Update:Increasing Mortality Calls For Action. Global Hepatitis Report 2017 pp 8. ISBN 978-92-4-156545-5

3. Hunt Richard: "Hepatitis Virus". University Of Southern California, Department Of Pathology and Microbiology, 2008-03-13.

4. Locarnini S 2004 . "Molecular Biology of Hepatitis B Virus". Semin. Liver Dis. 24 (Suppl 1): 3-10.

5. World Health Organization. Hepatitis B Fact Sheet No. 204. 2009. Available at http://www.who.int/csr/disease/hepatitis

6. National Heart, Lung, and Blood Institute (NHLBI). "How Is Sickle Cell Disease Diagnosed?". June 12, 2015. Archived from the original on 24 March 2016. Retrieved 8 March 2016.

7. National Human Genome Research Institute (NHGRI) "Learning about Sickle Cell Disease". May 9 2016.

8. Rees, DC. Williams, TN. Gladwin MT. (Sickle Cell Disease). Lancet. 386 (9757): 2018-31

9. GBD 2015: Disease and Injury Incidence and Prevalence, Collaborators. (8 October 2016). "Global,regional, and national incidence, prevalence, and years lived with disability for 310 diseases and injuries, 1990-2015: a systematic analysis for the Global Burden of Disease Study 2015". Lancet. **388** (10053): 1545–1602..

10. Lebby R (1846). "Case of Absence of The Spleen". Southern J of Med Pharmacol.

11. Mehdi Nouraie., Sergi Nekhai., Victor R Gordeuk. Sickle Cell Disease is associated with HIV but higher HBV and HCV Co morbidities In US Hospital Discharge Records. Sexually Transmitted Infections.2012;88:528-533).2012;88:528-533).
12. Fashola FA, Odaibo GN Aken'Ova YA, Olaleye OD: 'Hepatitis B and C viral markers in patients with sickle cell disease in Ibadan Nigeria'. African Journal of Medicine and Medical Sciences 2003; 32:293-5).

13. Omeje KN, Ibekwe RC, Ojukwu JO, Una AF, Ibe BC: Risk factors for hepatitis B surface antigenaemia among secondary school students in Abakaliki, South Eastern Nigeria. Niger J Paediatr 2017; 44 (1): 14 –21
14. Emeche GO Emodi IJ Ikefuna AN Ilechukwu GC Igwe WC Ejiofor OS Ilechukwu CA. Hepatitis B Infection In Nigeria – A Review. Niger Med J 2009; 50:18-22.

15. Akinbami, A.A.; Oshinaike, O.O.; Dosunmu, O.A.; Adeyemo, T.A.; Adediran, A.; Akanmu, S.; Wright, K.O.; Ilori, S.; Aile, K. Seroprevalence of Hepatitis B E

Antigen (Hbe Antigen) and B Core Antibodies (Igg anti-HBcore and IgM anti-HBcore) among Hepatitis B Surface Antigen Positive Blood Donors at a Tertiary Centre in Nigeria. BMC Res. Notes. 2012, Mar 28, 5, 167. DOI: 10.1186/1756-0500-5-167.

16. Bakarey **AS,** Ifeorah IM, Adewumi MO, Faleye TOC, Akere A, et al. (2017) Profiles of Hepatitis B Virus Serological Markers among Asymptomatic Population in Anambra State, Southeastern Nigeria. J Virol Antivir Res 6:3.

17. Gerlich WH (2013) Medical Virology of Hepatitis B: how it began and where we are now. Virol J 10: 1-25

18. Chu CM, Liaw YF (November 2007). "Predictive factors for reactivation of hepatitis B following hepatitis B e antigen seroconversion in chronic hepatitis B". Gastroenterology. **133** (5): 1458–65.

19. Forbi JC, Iperepolu OH, Zungwe T, Agwale SM. Prevalence of Hepatitis B e Antigen in Chronic HBV Carriers in North-Central Nigeria. J Health Popul. Nutr. 2012; 30(4): 377–382.

20. Milich D, Liang T, Jake. Exploring the Biologic Basis of Hepatitis B e Antigen in Hepatitis B Virus Infection. Hepatology 2003;38:1075–1086.DOI:10.1053/ jhep.2003.50453.

21. Ochola, E.; Ponsiono, O.; Orach, C.G.; Nankinga, Z.K.; Kalyango, J.N.; McFarland, W.; Karamagi, C. High Burden of Hepatitis B Infection in Northern Uganda: Resultof a Population – Based Survey. BMC Public Health. 2013, 13, 727. DOI: 10.1186/1471- 2458-13-727.

22. Bolarinwa Rahman A, Aneke John C, Olowookere Samuel A, Salawu Lateef: Seroprevalence of transfusion transmissible viral markers in sickle cell disease patients and healthy controls in Ile-Ife, South-Western Nigeria: A case–control study. J Applied Haematol (2015) 6(4): 162-167

23. Nsiah K. 1, Dzogbefia V.P. 1, Osei-Akoto A. 2, Ansong D. 2 Journal of Hematological Malignancies, March 2012, Vol. 2, No. 1

24. Samuel S. Antwi-Baffour, Kwadwo Adarkwah-Yiadom, Ransford Kyeremeh, David Nana Adjei, Mahmood S. Abdulai, Patrick F. Ayeh- Kumi. 'Incidence of Hepatitis B Surface Antigen among Sickle Cell Disease Patients Receiving

Transfusion Therapy'. International Journal of Biomedical Science and Engineering. Vol. 2, No. 1, 2014, pp. 7-10. doi: 10.11648/j.ijbse.20140201.12

25. Ampofo W, Nii-Trebi N, Ansah J, Abe K, Naito H, Aidoo S.et al. Prevalence of Blood- Borne Infectious Diseases in Blood Donors in Ghana. J Clin Microbiol (2002) 40(9): 3523-3525.

26. Chamberland M, Alter HJ, Busch MP, Nemo G, Ricketts M (2001). Emerging infectious disease in blood safety. Emerg. Infect. Dis; 7: 552-3.

27. Stephan Schaefer: Hepatitis B virus genotypes in Europe. Hepatology Research. (2007) Volume37, Issues1, Pages S20-S26. https://doi.org/10.1111/j.1872-034X.2007.00099

28. Hadziyannis SJ, Vassilopoulos: Immunopathogenesis of hepatitis B e antigen negative chronic hepatitis B infection. Antiviral Res. 2001 Nov;52(2):91-8.

29. Schillie S, Murphy TV, Sawyer M, Ly K, Hughes E, Jiles R, de Perio MA, Reilly M, Byrd K, Ward JW (20 December 2013). "CDC Guidance for Evaluating Health-Care Personnel for Hepatitis B Virus Protection and for Administering Postexposure Management". MMWR. Recommendations and reports : Morbidity and Mortality Weekly Report. Recommendations and reports / Centers for Disease Control. 62 (RR-10): 1–19.

30. Fasola Foluke Atinuke., Fadimu Patricia Adedoyin, Akpan Victoria Oluwabunmi: A Seven Year Review of the Seroprevalence of Transfusion Transmitted Infections in a Hospital Based Blood Bank in Ibadan, Nigeria Clinical Medicine Research 2017; 6(1): 1-8

Profiles of Hepatitis B Virus Serological Markers among Asymptomatic Population in Anambra State, Southeastern Nigeria *

Bakarey AS, Ifeorah IM et al

Abstract

Hepatitis B Virus (HBV) infection is apparent in endemic countries affecting millions of people. Further, the asymptomatic nature of the pathogen is a major public health concern. This study was designed to assess the burden of HBV by exploring the serologic markers of infection among consenting asymptomatic community dwellers in two cities in southeastern Nigeria.

A total of 405 blood specimens were tested for HBsAg, anti-HBs, HBeAg, anti-HBe, total anti-HBc and anti-HBc-IgM using ELISA technique. Overall, 14(3.5%) of the participants had detectable HBsAgout of which 1(7.1%) had HBeAg and 13 anti-HBe. Two of the HBsAg positives (14.3%) had detectable anti-HBc-IgM. A total of 144 (35.5%) had detectable anti-HBc, even as 65(57.0%) of them had the marker as the only serologic evidence of HBV exposure. Thirty-seven (9.1%) participants had anti-HBs only although all of them were borne before the start of the childhood HBV vaccination. Altogether, 224 (57.3%) had no detectable serological markers of HBV infection or immunity and were obviously at risk of HBV infection.

This study described various patterns of HBV serologic markers of infection in the study population and probable risk of virus spread. Our results support the need for urgent intervention and implementation of measures to control the spread of HBV infection in Nigeria.

*Bakarey AS, Ifeorah IM, Adewumi MO, Faleye TOC, Akere A, et al. (2017) Profiles of Hepatitis B Virus Serological Markers among Asymptomatic Population in Anambra State, Southeastern Nigeria. J Virol Antivir Res 6:3. doi: 10.4172/2324-8955.1000174

Keywords: HBV; Serological markers; Asymptomatic; Community dwellers; ELISA; Anambra; Nigeria

INTRODUCTION

Hepatitis B virus (HBV) infection is one of the most common infectious diseases of the world and has infected 2 billion people globally; leaving an estimated 248 million as chronic carriers [1,2]. Infection with HBV may lead to acute or chronic conditions with consequences such as liver cirrhosis and hepatocellular carcinoma (HCC) overtime. It has been estimated that 70 – 90% of the population with chronic HBV infection have normal liver function [3,4]. This group of people are said to be apparently healthy HBsAg carriers (asymptomatic) forming major component parts of the general population in endemic countries of Africa [5,6].Due to its largely asymptomatic nature, chronic viral hepatitis is a silent epidemic, and most people are unaware of their infection.

Epidemiological studies carried out in different parts of the world show that the characteristics of the population, such as sanitary conditions, lifestyle, hygiene, risk and socioeconomic factors are related to large variations in the frequency and prevalence of HBV infection[7,8].The major route of transmission of HBV in endemic regions like Nigeria is perinatal from Hepatitis B e Antigen (HBeAg)-positive mothers or through early horizontal transmission from close contacts with immediate family members[5,9]. However, this virus can also be spread via the use of contaminated blood and blood products, organs transplant from infected donors and unprotected sexual intercourse with an infectious person. Significantly, hepatitis B is a vaccine preventable infection, and WHO has recommended vaccination for several population groups ranging from infants to high risk adults.[10]

Hepatitis B virus has different serological markers of infection which include Hepatitis B surface antigen (HBsAg) and its corresponding antibody (anti-HBs), antibody to HBcAg (anti-HBc), Hepatitis B e antigen (HBeAg) and antibody to HBeAg (anti-HBe) **[11,12]**. Precisely, HBsAg beyond six (6) months of first detection, is a marker of chronic Hepatitis B infection[13], while, presence of anti-HBs demonstrates immunity to HBV either by vaccination or via resolved infection by the virus. Further, presence of antibody to the core antigen indicates an exposure to HBV irrespective of whether it is a recent or resolved infection [14]. It is possible to establish the infection or immunity status of a person in routine diagnostics with these three markers [12].Additionally, HBeAg correlates with the virus infectivity and the risk of progression to cirrhosis in chronic carriers, while its corresponding antibody often connotes less infectious state[13].

Due to the fact that HBV infection is associated with either one or multiples of these serological markers and this signifies different phases or stages of the infection [12] we therefore aimed in this study to assess the prevalence of ongoing or resolved HBV infection by investigating various serological markers among asymptomatic community dwellers of Anambra State in southeastern Nigeria.

METHODOLOGY

2.1 Study location

This cross-sectional community-based study was carried out at Onitsha and Nnewi communities in Anambra State. The two communities serve as commercial nerve centers of the state with people trouping in daily for business activities from neighboring towns, villages and states across the country. Population of these cities during the business hours is usually more than ten times of the residents, thus, making it difficult to ascertain the exact population. Apart from Christianity which

17

is the major religion in the area, some residents are adherents of African Traditional Religion (ATR). Apart from Ibo, the native language, many residents communicate in Pidgin English. These communities can boast of good health care facilities from which the residents and emigrants from neighboring communities and towns benefit from.

2.1.1 Enrolment of participants

A total of 405 consenting participants (M=194, F=211; age ranged 15-70 years and median age=26.4 years) were enrolled for the study in August, 2013. The study relied upon availability of participants in their houses, workplace and willingness to be involved in the study. The main assumption for using this approach was based on the premise that the target population is homogeneous and is likely to share similar characteristics and life style. Health education messages relating to HBV prevalence and prevention were provided to each prospective participant prior to their enrolment in the study. Subsequently, a structured questionnaire was used to capture the socio-demographic information of the target population. Blood sample was collected from each consenting participant by a trained phlebotomist. Ethical approval for the study was granted by the Anambra State Ministry of Health, Awka (MH/PHD/MISC/1). All the participants were well informed on the nature, purpose and processes involved in the study prior to their enrolment. Participation was voluntary while the non consenting participants were excluded from the study thereby maintaining the principle of autonomy. Verbal consent was used to enroll the participants into the study. Confidentiality, privacy and anonymity of the information for each participant were guaranteed for the sample provided.

2.1.2 Sample collection

Five milliliters of blood was collected from each participant by venipuncture. The blood sample was then dispensed into an appropriately labeled sterile container without any preservative or anticoagulant. Subsequently, the samples were transported to the laboratory at about 4-8°C in a cooler with frozen ice packs. Serum was separated from other blood components by low-speed centrifugation at 500g for 5 minutes and subsequently removed using a sterile disposable pipette. Two aliquots from each serum were made per sample in labeled sterile cryovials and stored at −20°C until ready for analysis. Laboratory analysis was carried out in the Department of Virology, and the Institute for Advanced Medical Research and Training, College of Medicine, University of Ibadan, Ibadan, Nigeria.

ELISA screening for HBV serological markers

All 405 samples were screened for HBsAg, anti-HBs, HBeAg, anti-HBe, total anti-HBc and anti-HBc-IgM using Enzyme Linked Immunosorbent Assay (ELISA) test kits (Diagnostic Automation/Cortez Diagnostic, California, USA). All assays were carried out according to manufacturer's instructions while the optical density was read using the Emax endpoint ELISA microplate reader (Molecular Devices, California, USA) and the results interpreted accordingly.

RESULTS

Overall, 14(3.5%) of the participants had detectable HBsAgout of which 1(7.1%) had HBeAg and 13 anti-HBe. Two of the HBsAg positives (14.3%) had detectable anti-HBc-IgM. In all, 144 (35.5.8%) of the participants had detectable total anti-HBc, while anti-HBs was detected in 97 (24.0%) (Tables 1 and 2).

The participants were subsequently grouped into 2 serological profiles: A (HBsAg positive) and B (HBsAg negative) (Figures 1 and 2). Profile A was subdivided into

3 subgroups, and B into 5 subgroups based on serologic markers present. Only one patient within profile A had detectable anti-HBc and HBeAg, thus, she was categorized as subgroup A1. A total of 12 patients with anti-HBe and anti-HBc were categorized as subgroup A2 while 1 participant with anti-HBc, anti-HBe and anti-HBs was categorized as A3. Within profile B, 130(33.2%) of the 391 HBsAg negative participants had anti-HBc. Among these 130 were 6(15.3%) subjects with detectable anti-HBc and anti-HBe who were categorized in subgroup B1. Sixty-five participants with anti-HBc only (16.6 %) were categorized into subgroup B2; and 59 others (15.1 %) with anti-HBs, anti-HBc and or without anti-HBe as B3. Subgroup B4 has 37 participants with detectable anti-HBs only, while 224 other participants without any detectable HBV serological markers categorized as B5 (Figure 2).

Serological profiles of HBV infection by age shows highest (62.8%) susceptibility for HBV infection (B5) among age groups31-40years while lowest rate (41.5%) among age group >50years. Highest rates for detectable isolated anti-HBs in profile B4 (25.0%) were observed in age groups<20years. Profile B3 had highest and lowest rates (21.6% and 5.1%) among age groups 41-50 and <20 years respectively. Also, highest rate (39.6%) for profile B2 was recorded in age group >50years and the lowest (2.6%) amongst 21-30years. Profile A (HBsAg-positive) with the majority categorized into A2 recorded highest rate (6.2%) in age group 31-40years and the lowest (1.8%) in 41-50years (Table 2).

Table 1: Distribution of serological markers of HBV infection by age among residents in Anambra State, Nigeria

Age Range (yrs)	No Tested	HBsAg (%)	HBeAg (%)	Anti-HBe (%)	Anti-HBc (%)	Anti-HBc-IgM (%)	Anti-HBs (%)
<20	39	0(0.0)	0(0.0)	0(0.0)	4(10.3)	0(0.0)	11(28.2)
21-30	129	4(3.1)	1(25.0)	9(7.0)	40(31.0)	1(25.0)	30(23.3)
31-40	129	9(7.0)	0(0.0)	13(10.1)	46(35.7)	1(11.1)	25(19.4)
41-50	55	1(1.8)	0(0.0)	3(5.5)	24(43.6)	0(0.0)	17(30.9)
>50	53	0(0.0)	0(0.0)	0(0.0)	30(56.6)	0(0.0)	14(26.4)
Total	405	14(3.5)	1(7.1)	25(6.2)	144(35.5)	2(14.3)	97(24.0)

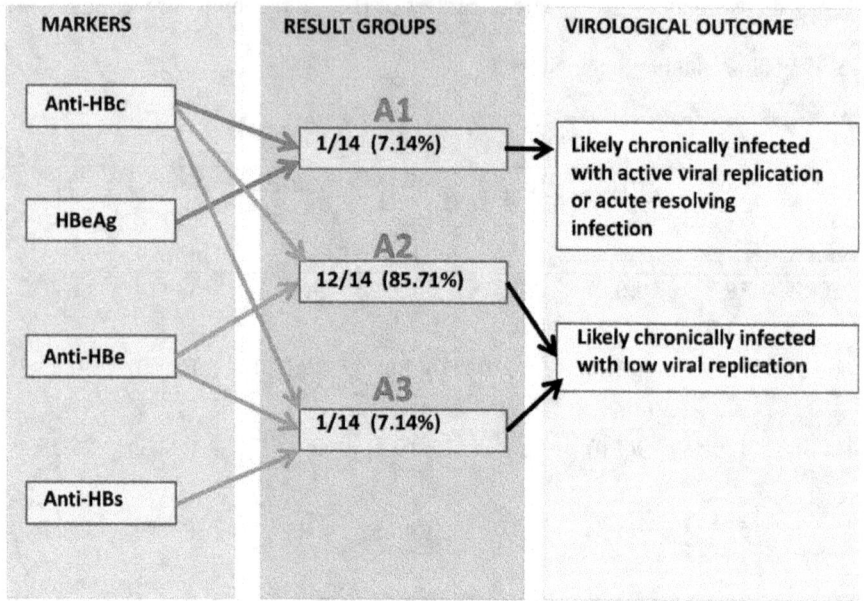

Figure 1: Profile A: Serological profile of HBsAg positive participants in the two communities in Anambra state ,Nigeria

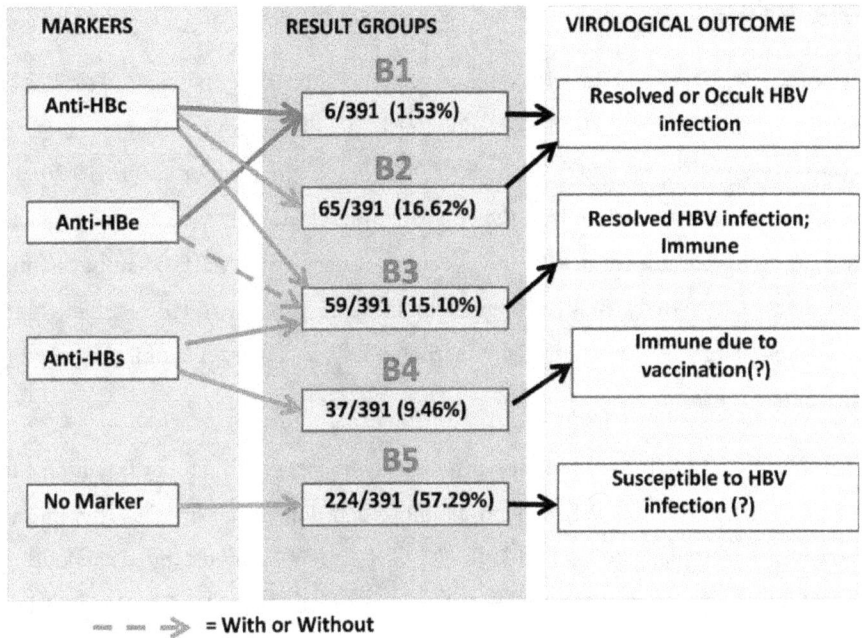

Figure 2 : Profile B: serological profiles of HBsAg Negative participants in the two communities in Anambra state Nigeria

DISCUSSION

An overall rate of 3.5% for HBsAg observed among the study population (Table 1) is within the range of 1.1%-4.3%previously reported from different parts of Nigeria[15,16,17], but lower than the 5.7%-12.3% range reported [18,19,20] in southern and northern regions of the country. Many factors may be adduced for the difference in rates, nevertheless, the overall prevalence of 3.5% HBs-antigenaemia detected in this study may not represent the true picture of HBV infection in southwest Nigeria considering the earlier findings reported from this region [21,22].

The rate of 7.1% (1/14) for HBeAg found in this study (Figure 1) is within the range of 6.4- 8.9% [6,8,9,16] found among blood donors in Nigeria. This rate is however lower than 26.7% (4/15) and 30.3% (10/33) reported by Anaedobe *et al.*[7] and Bayo *et al.*, [23] among other cohorts, respectively. The HBeAg has been described both as an indicator of active HBV replication, and as an immunomodulator that reduces the capability of children born to HBsAg and HBeAg positive mothers to clear the virus, thus making them chronic carriers and consequently, reservoirs of HBV in different populations [24].The participant with profile A1 tends to be highly infectious with active viral replication, since HBeAg is a marker of high infectivity[24,25]. He also poses a high risk of possible transmission not only to his sexual partners but to his household.

The 11 of the 12 participants in profile A2 (Figure 1) could be casesof chronic infection with low viral titers. Presence of anti-HBe may suggest good prognosis and is indicative of controlled viral replication in these individuals in profile A2, since persons with anti-HBe tend to have lower viraemia [25]. One might assume that patients in this subgroup are mostly inactive carriers, and thus may not

24

transmit the infection to others. However, mutations in the regions of the viral genome that codes for HBeAg can result in absence or decreased levels of detectable HBeAg, but this may not alter the sequeale of chronic infection[13It has been reported that HBeAg-negative HBV mutants prevail in the general populationof HBV carriers [26]. One of these 12 participants in profile A2 (Figure 1) was also positive for anti-HBc-IgM, thus, might be a case of acute infection. However, several studies have shown that many patients with chronic hepatitis B have low to moderate titers of anti-HBc-IgM [27], especially during acute exacerbation of chronic HBV infection [28].

In profile A3 is a participant with both HBsAg and anti-HBs serologic markers. This may be a case of chronic HBV infection as previous report has shown that in less than 1% of times chronic HBV carriers can be positive for both HBsAg and its corresponding antibody and has suggested that such patients be categorized as infectious [14]. Anti-HBs in absence of HBsAg indicates protection against HBV and may be acquired either through infection or vaccination [12]. Although, vaccinated individuals with anti-HBs are protected against clinical apparent hepatitis B, asymptomatic breakthrough infection in vaccinated population has been demonstrated [29].The presence of HBsAg in this participant could theoretically also portray breakthrough infection but vaccination and pre-existing anti-HBs are not known for this person. It is more likely that this is a chronic HBV carrier with a detectable but insufficient anti-HBs [30] response. It is worth mentioning that though breakthrough infections caused by immune escape mutants have been demonstrated, they have not been shown to represent a major problem yet [31,32].Further, the qualitative presence of anti-HBs alone after vaccination is not enough to confer HBV immunity as the titer must be up to 10mIU/mL. The levels might drop to less after 5 to 10 years post vaccination [33]and may need booster doses.

The 71 members of profiles B1 and B2 (Figure 2) could possibly be in the window period in which anti-HBs is yet to develop but have cleared the HBsAg below detectable limit of the test kit [34], however, they could also be candidates for occult HBV infection. Studies have shown that individuals with detectable anti-HBc with or without anti-HBs but negative for HBsAg can be viraemic at a low level [35,36,37].However, the majority of HBV particles in occult infected subject is not infectious[38].The rate of isolated anti-HBc(B2) recorded among those who were exposed to HBV was 57.0 % (65/114)(Figure 2). Isolated anti-HBc may represent resolved infection with the loss of anti-HBs, occult chronic HBV infection with levels of HBsAg below detectable limit, or a false positive reaction [39].It has been suggested that such individuals be regarded as non-immune to HBV and should be considered for vaccination.

Thirty-seven of the total 391(9.5%) HBsAg negative participants had detectable anti-HBs (B4), with highest rate in age group <20 years. This may be due to unspecific reaction since childhood HBV immunization started in 2004 in Nigeria, thus these adult population may not have benefitted from the program. On the other Anti-HBs alone without previous vaccination seems to be relatively frequent.

This study found a rate of 57.3% (224/405) of the population belonging to subgroup B5 (Figure 2 and Table 2) with no detectable marker to confirm previous exposure to HBV infection or vaccination.Thus, are at risk of being infected, they therefore are of public health concern to successful control of HBV infection, since if infected could transmit the virus.

Conclusion

This study described various HBV serological markers of infection among the study population and their virological significance. Our results confirm the need for urgent intervention and implementation of measures to control the circulation of HBV infection in Nigeria.

REFERENCES

1. Dény P. and Zoulim F (2010) Hepatitis virus: From diagnosis to treatment. PatholBiol (Paris),58: 245-253.
2. 2.Luo Z, Li L, and Ruan B(2012)Impact of the implementation of a vaccination strategy on hepatitis B virus infections in China over a 20-year period. International Journal of Infectious Diseases 16: e82–e88.
3. Ocama P, Opio C.K and Lee W.M (2005) Hepatitis B virus infection. Current status," The American Journal of Medicine 118:1413.e15-1413.e22,.
4. Wang F, Fan J, Zhang Z, Gao B et al (2014) The Global Burden of Liver Disease. Hepatology 60 -(6):2099-108
5. Ijeoma S, Nwokediuko S .Onyenekwe   B and Ijoma C (2009) Low Prevalence of Hepatitis "E" Antigen in Asymptomatic Adult Subjects with Hepatitis B Virus Infection in Enugu, South East Nigeria.The Internet Journal of Gastroenterology 10:1.
6. Japhet M.O , Adesina O.A, Donbraye E and Adewumi M.O (2011) Hepatitis B core IgM antibody (anti-HBcIgM) among hepatitis B surface antigen (HBsAg) negative blood donors in Nigeria .Virol J 8: 513.
7. Anaedobe C.G , Fowotade A , Omoruyi C.E and Rasheed Ajani Bakare (2015) Prevalence, socio-demographic features and risk factors of Hepatitis

B virus infection among pregnant women in Southwestern Nigeria. Pan Afr Med J . 20 : 406.

8. OluyinkaO.O , Tong H.V, Bui Tien S et al (2015) Occult Hepatitis B Virus Infection in Nigerian Blood Donors and Hepatitis B Virus Transmission Risks. PLoS One 10:7.

9. Lavanchy D (2005)Worldwide epidemiology of HBV infection, disease burden, and vaccine production. J. ClinVirol. 34,Suppl1,pp.Si-S3,2005

10.UNAIDS report on global AIDS epidemic 2012.Geneva, 2012.

11..Lok A.S, Lai C.L and Wu P.U (1988) Prevalence of isolated antibody to hepatitis B core antigen in an area endemic for hepatitis B virus infection: implications in hepatitis B vaccination programs. Hepatology 8: 766–70.

12.Gerlich W.H (2013) Medical Virology of Hepatitis B: how it began and where we are now . Virology Journal 10(239): 1-25.

13.Krajden M, McNabb G and Petric M (2005) The Laboratory diagnosis of hepatitis B virus. Can J Infect Dis Med microbial 16(2): 65-72.

14.Dufour D.R , Lott J.A, Nolte F,S et al. (2000) Diagnosis and monitoring of hepatic injury.I.Performance characteristics of laboratory tests. ClinChem 46:.2027-2049,.

15.Ochola E, Ocama P, Orach C.G, Nankinga Z K, Kalyango J.N et al (2013) High burden of Hepatitis B Infection In Northern Uganda: result of a population based survey. BMC Public Health 13:727.

16.Aba HO and Aminu M (2016) Seroprevalence of hepatitis B virus serological markers among pregnant Nigerian women. Ann AfrMed 15(1):20-7

17..BakareyA S, Ifeorah I.M, FaleyeT.O.C,Adewumi M.O,Akere A et al (2017) Hepatitis B Virus Serological Markers in a Rural Community in Southeastern Nigeria.British Journal of Medicine and Medical Science

21(1):1-9.

18. Akani C.I, Ojule A.C, OpurumH.C ,Ejilemele A.A (2005) Sero-prevalence of hepatitis B surface antigen (HBsAg) in pregnant women in Port Harcourt, Nigeria. Niger Postgrad Med J,12 (4) : 266-70.

19. Olaleye O.A, Kuti O, MakindeN.O,UjahA.O,Olaleye O.A et al (2013) Perinatal transmission of hepatitis B virus infection in Ile-Ife, South Western, Nigeria. J Neonatal Perinatal Med 6(3) : 231-236.

20. FaleyeT.O.C, Adewumi M.O, Ifeorah I.M, OmoruyiC.E,Bakarey A.S (2015b) Detection and Circulation of Hepatitis B virus Immune Escape Mutants among Asymptomatic Community dwellers in Ibadan, southwestern Nigeria. Int J Infect Dis 2416: 1-8.

21. Okonko I, Okerentugba P, Innocent A.H (2012) Detection of Hepatitis B Surface Antigen (HBsAg) Among Children In Ibadan, Southwestern Nigeria,"Int J Infect Dis 10: 10-12.

22. Udeze A.O ,Aliyu A.S, KolawoleM,Okonko O, Sule W.F (2012) Hepatitis B surface antigenaemia and risk factors of transmission among apparently healthy students of university of Ilorin, Ilorin-Nigeria. SciAfr 11:1-8.

23. Bayo P, Ochola E, Oleo C and Nwaka D.A (2014) High prevalence of Hepatitis B virus infection among pregnant women attending anti-natal care: a cross sectional study in Northern Uganda. BMJ Open (4) :11.

24. Stevens C, Beasley R, Tsui J and Lee W.C(1975) Vertical transmission of hepatitis B antigen in Taiwan. N Engl J Med 292:771-774.

25. Milich D and Liang T.J (2003) Exploring the biologic basis of of Hepatitis B e Antigen in Hepatitis B virus infection. Hepatology 38:1075-1086.

26. Forbi J.C, Iperepolu O.H, Zungwe T, Agwele S.M (2012) Prevalence of hepatitis B e antigen in chronic HBV carriers in North-central Nigeria," J Health PopulNutr 30 (4):377-382.

27. Gerlich W.H, Uy A., Lambrecht F and Thomssen.R (1986) Cutoff levels of immunoglobulin M antibody against viral core antigen for differentiation of acute,chronic and past Hepatitis B Virus infection. Journal of clinical Microbiology 24:288-293.

28. Puri P (2013) Acute Exacerbation of Chronic Hepatitis B: The Dilemma of Differentiation from Acute Viral Hepatitis B. Journal of Clinical and Experimental Hepatology 3 (4):301-312.

29. Stramer S.L, Wend U, Candotti D. Foster G.A,Hollinger F.B et al. (2011) Nucleic acid testing to detect HBV infection in blood donors. New Engl J Med (364):236-247.

30. Gerlich WH. (2007) The enigma of concurrent hepatitis B surface antigen (HBsAg) and antibodies to HBsAg. Clin Infect Dis. 2007 May 1;44(9):1170-2. Epub 2007 Mar 19

31. Chang M (2010) Breakthrough HBV infection in vaccinated children in Taiwan: surveillance for HBV mutants. Antiviral therapy 15:463-469.

32. Shao Z.J,Zhang L, XuJQf (2011) Mother to infant transmission of Hepatitis B virus :A Chinese experience. J Med virol 83:791-795.

33. .Mahoney F.J (1999) Update on diagnosis, management and prevention of hepatitis B virus infection. ClinMicrobiol Rev 12:351-366.

34. Tong S, JisuL,Wands J.R et al (2013) Hepatitis B virus genetic variants :biological properties and clinical implications. Emerging Microbes and Infections l2: 10.

35. Manzini P, Girotto M, Borsotti R et al (2007) Italian blood donors with antiHBc and occult hepatitis B virus infection. Haematologica 92:1664-1670.

36. SatakeM,Taira R, Yugi H et al(2007) Infectivity of blood components with low hepatitis B virus DNA levels identified in a lookback program. Transfusion 47:1197–1205.

37. Bouike Y, Imoto S ,.Mabuchi O et al (2011) Infectivity of HBV DNA positive donations identified in look-back studies in Hyogo-Prefecture, Japan. Transfus Med 21:107-115.

38. Allain J.P, Hewitt P E, Tedder R.S et al (1999) Evidence that antiHBc but not HBV DNA testing may prevent some HBV transmission by transfusion. Br J Haematol 107:186–95.

39. Walz A, S. Wirth,J. Hucke et al (2009) Vertical Transmission of Hepatitis B Virus (HBV)from Mothers Negative for HBV Surface Antigen and Positive for Antibody to HBV Core Antigen. The Journal of Infectious Diseases 200: 1227–1231,2009.

Contents

Publisher: Eliva Press SRL

Email: info@elivapress.com

Eliva Press is an independent publishing house established for the publication and dissemination of academic works all over the world. Company provides high quality and professional service for all of our authors.

Our Services:
Free of charge, open-minded, eco-friendly, innovational.

-All services are free of charge for you as our author (manuscript review, step-by-step book preparation, publication, distribution, and marketing).
-No financial risk. The author is not obliged to pay any hidden fees for publication.
-Editors. Dedicated editors will assist step by step through the projects.
-Money paid to the author for every book sold. Up to 50% royalties guaranteed.
-ISBN (International Standard Book Number). We assign a unique ISBN to every Eliva Press book.
-Digital archive storage. Books will be available online for a long time. We don't need to have a stock of our titles. No unsold copies. Eliva Press uses environment friendly print on demand technology that limits the needs of publishing business. We care about environment and share these principles with our customers.
-Cover design. Cover art is designed by a professional designer.
-Worldwide distribution. We continue expanding our distribution channels to make sure that all readers have access to our books.

www.elivapress.com